Praise for *to li...*

"Discussing *to linger on hot co...* phor. These are poems forged in ...ru beauty. They burn with the truth of detail, making poetical the unspeakable experience of losing a child. To gaze into these flames is to find solace, connection and the authentic voices of survival and inspiration."

—Vanessa Gorman, Filmmaker
Losing Layla

"Raw, evocative, compelling. A heartfelt tumble down the rabbit hole of child loss into a world that is frequently hidden, often taboo but ultimately needs to be exposed. *to linger on hot coals* shines a light on the reality of the "other" family tree — the one with gnarled tree trunks and missing branches that so many mothers invisibly carry every day. A collective of hearts and souls that beat even in the ashes, and breathe life into the unseen."

—Pia Dorer, Producer/Director/Editor
It's Not All Black and White

"The gift of this collection is truth. The truth that ranges from vivid and raw to quiet and numb, all of it equally true. *to linger on hot coals* is the words of many writers unknown to me somehow revealing my story. It is like reading the sounds of my heart and the voice in my head over the past eleven years since I came to know the cold truth of death before life. And yet it is also the tapestry of warm comfort that affirms who we are as changed beings and reminds us we are never alone."

—Carrie Fisher-Pascual, Executive Producer
The STILL Project

"These poems sing, dance, scream, sigh, and honor as mothers parent the legacy of their children by giving voice to the continuing love for the babies no longer on this earth."

—Nina Bennett, Author
Forgotten Tears A Grandmother's Journey Through Grief and *Sound Effects*

"While words can never fully capture the magnitude of the loss a mother feels when her baby dies, this collection of poems gives expression to our grief and thus makes us feel less alone. This anthology is also a sweet reminder of the depths of our love for the children who will live on in our hearts forever."
—Carol Cirulli Lanham, PhD, Author
Pregnancy After a Loss: A Guide to Pregnancy After a Miscarriage, Stillbirth, or Infant Death

"These poems… will validate the experience for so many who are struggling with their loss. This book will help narrow that crevasse between a grieving mother's head and her heart as she learns how to go on living after the loss of her baby."
—Patti Anewalt, PhD, LPC, FT
Director at Pathways Center for Grief & Loss

"*to linger on hot coals* is raw and healing. …these words flowed from the pages like music for my broken spirit. I would recommend it to friends who don't know how to help, family who wish they could take our pain away, and the families who will read this piece of art and find their own stories woven throughout."
—Larisa L. Barth, Founder
Held Your Whole Life

"A breathtaking collection of real, true, raw, exposed emotion. Never before have I felt so connected to so many amazing women at one time. We are not alone in our deep, penetrating sadness. Simply amazing."
—Bridget Crews, Founder
Molly Bears

to linger on hot coals

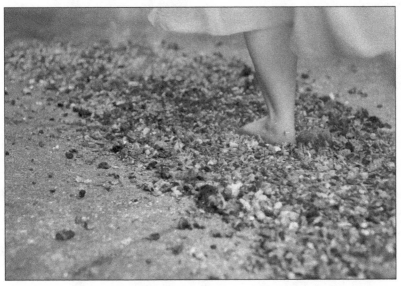

collected poetic works from grieving women writers

Stephanie Paige Cole
Catherine Bayly

Strategic Book Publishing and Rights Co.

Strategic Book Publishing and Rights Co.
12620 FM 1960, Suite A4-507
Houston, TX 77065
www.sbpra.com

ISBN: 978-1-62857-565-1

For Madeline
—SPC

For SSGB
—CAGB

Contents

Foreword

by Dr. Joanne Cacciatore

"I cannot live if she does not live."

Death. Death came. Death came into my body. Death came into my body and took my child. Death came into my body and took my child, leaving me in its carnage.

It was 1994. For ten long months we waited, all eyes turned toward me for the greatest performance of my life. Our bags were packed, laid across the top was her organic cotton sleeper with shiny silver snaps, embroidered in mint green thread, *"Going Home."*

I was no novice at pregnancy and birth, feeling overambitious bravado after three lip-splitting naturalis partus. Still, a quiescent sense of unease tugged at my arm. Dare I say it aloud? *"Something doesn't feel right."* The obstetrician advised me well: put your feet up, take a bath, and relax. I put my worry in a box, neatly, on the shelf in the closet next to my high school yearbook and old Peter Frampton concert tickets. *"Everything will be okay."* It was seeringly hot that summer day, my ankle bones hidden beneath swollen tissue, when labor pangs struck... .

And then, Death kicked in the door and violated me, right there, on the clean white sheets that smelled of bleach and teddy bears. He didn't kiss me. Or ask permission. Or even warn me. He just held me down and took her, the most precious and inviolable piece of me. Just like in the movies of near-death phenomena, I left my body. I floated on the

ix

ceiling, watching the slow-motion movements of men in white, frame by frame, as they put her lifeless eight-ebony-pounds-of-well-nourished-baby into my arms. I was stunned and disoriented. Three hours later, I crawled past the nursery toward the exit, empty-wombed and empty armed, a shamed outcast. She would not be 'going home' with me at all. The doctor lied. Her sleeper lied. I lied.

I wandered the aisles of the 24 hour Walgreens at 3 am looking for a pump to ease my gorging breasts, hot with fury. My uterus collapsed on itself, pregnant with unspeakable shock, grief, and despair. Her death became a blockbuster horror film I watched over and over- sounds, sights, smells, glances. The kind of terror-inducing movie you cannot possibly watch but from which you are unable to avert your gaze. I listened to the burning rationalizations of ministers and counselors and UPS drivers, like sage on the altar: *"All things happen for a reason," "You're young, you'll have more," "She just wasn't meant to be," "At least it wasn't one of your older children," "God has a plan for you,"* and *"Maybe something was wrong with her."* The world had shattered, language had no meaning, and my heart was eviscerated. I paced the hallways at night seeking her like a wild animal in captivity or an amputee searching for a missing limb. Every cell in my body craved her. I could not eat. Sleep. Think. Defend myself against an unsympathetic world. I could not care. I opened the russet envelope stamped "Office of Vital Records" that held her death certificate as proof of my failed performance. My Judas-body had not brought forth life. *"I cannot live if she does not live."* I was amongst the walking dead.

Indeed, in cultures around the world, childbirth is revered and celebrated as one of the most anticipated, emotionally charged of all human experiences. But sometimes, about one in 120 births, the baby dies. And this death is the ultimate paradox: Primal messages of birth, bonding, and maternal love coalesce with messages of death, departure, and insufferably traumatic grief.

Still, perhaps because of the systemic paternalization in childbirth, the process of recognition for babies stillborn has been a long and winding road. Two decades ago, the death of a baby to stillbirth was the dirty family secret, that which we dared not speak. Only one book, written nearly a decade earlier, would reach through the hands of time and provide a framework for this peculiarly painful state of hades: *Stillborn, The Invisible Death* by Dr. John DeFrain. But in 1994, the death of a baby to stillbirth was considered a reproductive or pregnancy loss, even a mere "adverse pregnancy outcome." Society dislikes truth: A baby, a loved and wanted child, died. Instead, these babies were dismissed as an asterisk, and grieving mothers' – and fathers'- experiences of loss were minimized and dismissed. These babies were not counted in infant mortality data (and still aren't), they were issued death certificates but not birth certificates (we started the movement to change this in 1998 and now more than three dozen states offer the option for a birth certificate), a dearth of research explored the lived experiences of families after baby death and what research did exist lumped stillbirth into studies about abortion and miscarriage rather than infant/child death, federal health funding initiatives did not include stillbirth in their funding agenda (we changed this in 2003), and these babies' lives were quickly glossed over as if they'd never existed, as if they'd never mattered. We lingered on hot coals.

But the unified voices of mothers and fathers and sisters and brothers and grandparents and caring professionals over the past two decades have shifted the tide for babies stillborn and their families. And the pressure for recognition, research, and competent psychosocial care has come full circle. We are silent no more. Rather, we are their voices. We are the voices that sing: *It is our time, it is their time.* It is time to speak their truth. It is time to speak grief's truth. It is time to speak love's truth, one which never dies and which will no longer be quelled.

To Linger on Hot Coals… yes, to linger is to burn, ravage, blister. And this collection of poetry, save the joie de vivre, is faithful to its title. It sings their songs with all the sharp notes of bitter verity. It is a collective purging, pleading, pardoning. It is anguish spilled onto many keyboards, contractions long into night hours, pangs until the poem is born, words created from each letter, giving form to that which is invisible, that which is the unmendable, albeit beautiful, wound. It will move you. It will seduce you into its darkness. It will take away your breath. It invites you into the space between self and other as Stephanie Cole's piece *For My Mother* does:

you did not touch
you did not move
you did not weep, though your heart must have shattered
your granddaughter dead
your own daughter dying before your eyes
and you, unable to move the mountains between
what we needed and
what we had

Or Angie Yingst's honest portrayal of death avoidance in *Of This We Shall Not Speak*:

You came into my home,
and did not speak of death.
But death was what we were doing...
You said that death talk made you uncomfortable.
And besides, you said, you wouldn't want to talk of death,
if your baby died.
I thought that I would call you again
when I could speak of something other than death.
I still think that some days.

Then, there is the longest journey back into ones self, into the place of unanswered questions, unreachable destinations, elusive concordance, and lurid acrimony as in the way Catherine Bayly's *Stillborn adj.* captures sublime anguish:

there, I found a moth pressed
between the pages, like its own
little translucent, ephemeral leaf,
with veins for words, and blood
drained out, and more years dead
than living, and through its forewing
I read (of an infant) born dead.

In what kind of world do children die before their parents? In what kind of world do children die before their birth? Anne Morris, in *The Physics of Losing You*, challenges a universe where babies can- and do- die.

An object at rest stays at rest.
The tiny circle of your heart, so still.
So still and silent that not even the force
of our prayers, our screams, our love,
our labor
could move you again.

Dear baby, breaking the laws of our universe.

And Hannah Logan Morris speaks of maternal love and remembrance *Every Morning* with her precious Joseph:

I
rubbed circles of lotion into my belly,
caressed my belly,
held it,
hugged it,
rested my hands on it,
gazed at it,
watched my profile in the mirror
growing...
I cradled you in one arm at night as I fell asleep.
And I sang to you every morning.

In a *furor sanandi* (rage to cure) world, intolerant of grief and its manifestations, we journey into the imminence and unpredictability of grief after a baby's death with Stephanie Cole's *Untitled II* and her own unhinging:

and then
five years later
you will sit in your car
in the dark
in the parking lot of Barnes & Noble
and you will put your forehead on the steering wheel
and you will cry
and you will cry
and you will cry

And cry we do.

Our children are stories waiting to be told. Our children are hearts waiting to be opened. Our children are great teachers waiting to be heard. Our children are poems waiting to be born. Our children are deserts waiting to be crossed, from Kara LC Jones, *It's all an experiment in free form*:

These are the things we find in the desert.
These are the ingredients of a life lived till death.
These are the frames in which we hang ourselves...
These are the boundaries we push by simply cheating
death each wide eyed morning.

Nearly two decades after I watched as they lowered her pink satin casket into the red earth, I feel her inhalations, resurrected in the songs of my sisters in mourning. I feel her exhalations, reborn in the movement toward recognition of these precious *children*. Stillbirth is a fundamental contradiction: a moment when life and death meet at the edge. And all these years later, I remember, well, those words *"I cannot live if she does not live."* Indeed, I did not live, not in the same way. I, like the mother-poets in this collection, was irreparably changed that fateful day. But in some small and meaningful way, *To Linger on Hot Coals* is their breath, their beating hearts, their mark in the world. And perhaps this is one step toward rebirth, for me, for her, for us, for them. And so, I live, she lives, we live. They live.

Joanne Cacciatore, PhD, LMSW
October, 2013
Sedona, Arizona
Arizona State University
MISS Foundation

Introduction

When this collection began as a seed in our minds—really, unofficially, from the moment our friendship began—we were both years away from losing our oldest children, our daughters. And today, as *to linger on hot coals* nears publication, the girls would be six and seven. We imagine them brunettes—the kinds of kids who dance, adventure, paint, and create, fitting into our hearts and houses like our living children. But, of course, they've been gone for years. And yet we've wondered aloud to each other, while picking fruit, whether we should *feel better than this*, whether *her hair was really brown*, whether *it will ever make sense for them to be this gone*.

This book grew from those musings, and our inabilities to tie neat bows around our family lives (however beautiful and many textured the ribbons). Through years, we've found ourselves in the relentless ebb and flow of grief, which any bereft person can relate to. So, we were both delighted and saddened when the poems for *to linger on hot coals* came rolling in. In truth, we contacted mostly poets we knew, asking them to share their work on losing their own children. So, unsurprisingly, the beauty of the contained poems left us breathless. But what stuck out for us was the constant repetition—the rise and fall structure also mirrored the grief we felt certain we'd never leave fully behind. Swells of peace at seeing children in peculiar sunsets, followed by massive shatters on mornings simply waking up to our babies still gone.

This pattern is inescapable and encapsulates the process of human loss. So, when organizing *to linger on hot coals*, we decided very quickly not to wrap the book up neatly. This would not be a straightforward journey, from the moment of loss to some peace-finding, although in some ways it is that too. Between those places, are fully jagged years and small, smooth stones of real beauty. When reading this book, we realize the reader—the ally, the grandmother, the newly bereft—may wish for a sweet film-style dénouement. But we beg you to resist that desire. Rather, we hope you will use this book as a tool for coming to grips with the power of loss (and perhaps love) over our writers' lives. Their impossible desire to create sacred things, raw and polished, out of mourning is at the heart of the journey. We hope this collection will help us all come nearer to peace with our grieving and the roles our children play in the stories we create.

When sifting through poems, we hoped a quickly shifting tone would give the collection a dual purpose. We see *to linger on hot coals* as a serious collection, full of precise language and lyric, as well as a piece of art that truly represents its bittersweet subject. In kind, some of the poems here are raw, written in the early days of our grief. And we hope they will gift the new parent with a sense of normalcy during those painful firsts. But, between those wrenching poems, are some impeccably crafted small birds of poems—the poems *lingering* nearly invisibly in each of us, so many years later. This book is for the mother who has just arrived home; the mother who has just picked up the pen and scratched her child's name; the mother who steps out again into a searing world and feels alone; and the mother who, years later, looks out over the cool ocean and smiles and chokes at once.

SPC & CAGB
September 2013

to linger on hot coals

I am changed.

Stephanie Paige Cole

blood from your body
has pulsed through my heart, my veins
of course I am changed.

Still Life

Catherine Bayly

I turn your photos at all angles.

Upside down, sideways, longways, backwards.
I try to get inside of them.
I try to touch your dimensions.
Today, you are really gone.
I miss you so much and my heart breaks.
It is not beautiful today.
It is not a sweet sadness.
It is frantic, and felt through gritted teeth.
In moments, I want to cry out the worst words.
But, I do it silently, mouth open, no sound.
You can't hear me say those things.
I pray (scream) you are watching me.
Knowing how much I miss you.
If I knew all along you would die,
I would be pregnant with you again.
Just to have those moments of holding you.
I would do it right.
I would kiss you like I kiss your sister.
In the soft hollow under the chin.
I would kiss and weep into the palms of your hands.
I would take beautiful photos.
I would know then what I know now.
That more than two years later,
It would hurt like it was yesterday.
That missing you would feel like
My organs ripped from my body.
Worse than that.

I would know that nothing feels worse.
I would know for sure that I would never be the same.
I would prepare for this agony.
I would drink in your soft skin.
I would remember your baby shoulders.
I would brush your long hair.
I would dress you so gently.
I would hold you until the nurse begged to take you away.
I would photograph you from all angles.
So that I could never forget the way your
Neck met your baby chest.
I would plaster my house with the pictures of you.
I would show them to everyone I meet.

Death

Hannah Logan Morris

I gave birth to death.

Our baby boy, stillborn. I gave birth to him knowing he had already died. Knowing all the labor, all the pain, would be for nothing. Wishing they could anesthetize me and cut him out and I could wake up a year later, another eight-month baby growing healthy in my womb.

But, delivery is indicated, they told me after showing me on the monitor where our baby's heart was hollow and still.

The drive to the hospital was like driving to my own funeral.

I gave birth to death.

But I gave birth. In the end, I know that going through it was the biggest gift to my son I could have given him. To be present, to be awake, to open up my body and let him go, was the only right way to honor his passing. I gave him life, carried him for eight months, and birthed him.

Stillbirth. It is still birth.

And still, I give birth to Death every day. Every day that I wake alive, I must acknowledge Death. To have our baby in my life, I must invite Death in, too.

What if Death is a woman? my wife asks.

4

On the eve of our baby's due date, 5 weeks after his birth, we decide to welcome Death into our lives.

What if Death is a woman? A woman who is simply doing her job. After all, it's a job someone has to do. She is older, stern but not unkind. Weathered, but unbowed by the weight of her task. Perhaps she weeps as she does her work. But she is unapologetic. Accepting.

I look this Death over. She holds our baby in her arms, partially wrapped in her cloak. Neither tender nor threatening. Was she a mother once, too?

I take one step closer.

She didn't snatch him away, I see. She came slowly, quietly. I came because I had to, she tells me.

I look Death in the eye.

I gave birth to you, I say.

And I say, Come in.

First published on Glow in the Woods, 4/22/13

Draped in Mythology

Kara LC Jones

She stood staring
into the bathroom mirror.
Her body felt different,
Mind rolled over
simple events
she'd paid no heed to...

retching when brushing her teeth,
fatigue in the heat of summer,
inability to walk to town
without feeling asphyxiated

Her body felt draped
in a mythology she could not understand.
She did not understand
the mirror image staring back at her.

Stepping back,
she felt the world slip away from her.
A thick, red velvet cape
surrounded her as the unfathomable happened:

blood and body
began its escape
covering the floor,
flooding the bath,
seeping into the ground
beneath the blooming flowers,
fading summer to fall.

6

Her body emptied itself,

princes
dragon's blood
ghosts of slain kings.

When the fully formed sac
found its way to the dirt and seed,
she felt consumed
by earth and worms,
the very beings who would
reclaim her fallen prince,

and she ached.

She returned to the mirror.
It was not the fairest of all reflected.
Rather the show was
an echo of grief,
an empty clay pot.

And when the rains came,
she was forced to
let go the physical,

nothing left

but the
draping of a mythology

she did not want to understand.

Inspired by the book Walking on Alligators

Expecting
Laura Seftel

It is an indelible loss — like ink on a white blouse,
something ruined, irreversible.
Bright red swirls in the morning waters.
You stare silently, you think it might be a dream,
a dream just before waking.

You're losing something but you can not stop it.
Your husband is running up the stairs.

Waiting for the doctor to phone
watching television blindly.
Not moving, so as not to stir things up, not to feel anything.
Thinking, perhaps this is the worst day of my life.

What they didn't tell you
is that it's not over in a minute, or even a half hour.
You will eat lunch in an Indian restaurant
and at an odd instant recall
you are having a miscarriage.

"It was never viable" the doctor explains.
You can't seem to hear her — you notice her kind eyebrows.
The nurses locate places for you to weep.
"Get my husband — I can't understand the doctor."
Tears springing, as if to wash away this wrong story.
Waiting for her to say there is still a baby somewhere.

I cannot find myself. Perhaps I have slipped out as well.
Perhaps something has broken open.

Something has been lost.
And now what to do with the prenatal vitamins?

The cherries on our tree, tiny hard miracles,
Have quickly turned over-ripe.
Sitting in metal bowls they exude their sticky juices.
There seem to be always more of them.
How will it end? How many pies can I bake?
My hands are already stained
with the work of slitting each one and
pulling out the stone.

Reprinted with permission from Seftel, L. (2006)
Grief Unseen: Healing Pregnancy Loss Through the Arts.
London: Jessica Kingsley Publishers.

For Christian

Carly Marie Dudley

A dimly lit hospital room.
A failing epidural.
Nausea, blasted nausea.
Mother groans and new born cries.
But there were to be no newborn cries in our room.

Pushing, breathing, pain, silence.
Deafening silence,
followed by a river of tears.
It was over.
Yet it was not.
The ending was only the beginning.

They separated you from me.
You were placed on my chest.
Instant love.
Intense heartache.

Breathe baby breathe.
Why won't you wake up?
Please baby.
Can you not stay with us?
I love you.
We love you.

She took you from me.
We left you in a hospital filled with baby ghosts.
Our hearts cracked wide open.
They burned your body down to ashes.

And the Winter of our grief set in.
We broke.

In between the whys and what ifs
I searched for you in sunsets and star filled skies.
I burned candles in memory of you.
Prayed to you.
Spoke of you.
Dreamed of you.
Lived and breathed you.
But you were not there.
You were nowhere to be found.
And so I lay in the darkness.
Without you.

Then one day,
I felt the warmth of the sun on my skin.
I thought I saw you in the field.
I found your spirit colouring the sunset.
I heard your cries in other babies.
My imagination was re awakened.
And you were reborn to me.
But you had never truly left me.
You were there the entire time.
I just could not see you,
for I cannot see my own heart.

For My Mother
Stephanie Paige Cole

you stayed there all night in that chair at the foot of my bed,
    a little off to the side
he slept on and off
cried on and off
I shook under piles of blankets
and dreamed up quiet ways to die
and you sat so still

you must have wanted to hold me, I'm sure
I remember now how you tried to tuck
my hair behind my ear
gently touch my arm
kiss my forehead
I blocked your every attempt to caress this body I had already
    dismissed as worthless
and what would you have felt if I had let you touch me
a cold heavy shell
empty except for the failure

you did not touch
you did not move
you did not weep, though your heart must have shattered
your granddaughter dead
your own daughter dying before your eyes
and you, unable to move the mountains between
what we needed and
what we had
and then it was time

he could not help me then, he could not
his soul was burning badly and his heart had fallen to the
    ground, too heavy to lift
he doubled over and his body shook with sadness
the depths of which are still too great to know
it must have hurt you to watch him
you must have wanted to scoop him up like a baby bird
broken wings and failing heart
run him frantic down the halls to his mother
but there was no time

you came to my side and held my leg and I did all there was
    left to do
brought her body to the surface so that we could say
    goodbye

and when she came, you were there
we couldn't look, but you did
your warm hands were the first to touch her sacred form
you washed her gently, so gently
and you did not cry, or if you did
you did so silently

you did not make her death about yourself

you dried her soft skin and wrapped her in a blanket
you handed her to her father
he handed her to me

you did for me what I could not do for her
you gave me life and helped me keep it
your hands still holding it today

Still.

Anne Morris

I sit motionless, draw inside,
duck my head
while the world goes hurtling past.
While all the objects of my universe orbit—
sickening circles—
while everything else keeps going.
I thought it was you who had stopped, but I have.

Still.

Your head, your hands,
your feet
under my hand
inside her womb.
Your mouth, your fingers,
your eyes that should be opening.

Still.

My mind races,
jumps, scans, launches.
I rush from car to office to school to house.
I offer my time, my help, my words.
I teach, explain,
find solace and exhaustion
in moving.

Still.

Your absence.
Her hand in the darkness.
The sun that seems still to orbit us.
My heart, opening to you.

Grief Is Labor in Reverse

Hannah Logan Morris

I am having another contraction.

Grief is labor in reverse.

It starts with a cry. Low, animal cries, coming from my throat. Our baby, our baby, our baby. Our baby is silent. Still.

A death, a birth. My heart dilates, bleeds, breaks open. The pain blurs memory. Those first few days no longer clear, but I can tell the story I've recreated.

We leave the hospital with empty arms. A false rewind, our bodies staggering backwards towards before. The house, half-ready for a baby. The stroller dismantled, repacked into the box. Receipts dug out, diaper bag and car seat and baby swing turned back into gift cards. Borrowed breast pump returned.

At first the contractions are close together. Every few seconds, wave upon wave of unbearable clenching and release.

Once that contraction is over, it's never coming back, the yoga teacher says. I breathe, trying to relax into it. Tears stream down my face. Once this one is over, it's never coming back. Never coming back.

These first few weeks out, we're allowed to scream and shout and rage. Too hot, too cold. Stop touching me. Get out of my face. No, come closer, hold me, touch me, rub there.

16

Anything is permissible. Our family and friends stand by, ready to run for the ice chips. Ready to run into our arms. Ready to call for help.

The contractions slow. A few minutes to catch my breath, a few hours. These moments in between are a strange relief. The eye of a hurricane. I know the winds are about to shift direction.

Change position.

We walk. We clean the house. We distract ourselves with TV and movies, podcasts, stories read aloud. We rock in the glider. We hold each other. We let the dishes pile up. We rearrange the furniture. We sit still. We walk.

The contractions begin to come further apart. Every other day. A contraction or two is no big fuss. No one jumps for the hospital bag. No one calls or texts the news. The sympathy cards go from three or four a day, to two, to one. Then an empty mailbox.

The contractions are more erratic now. No point in timing them. The literature speaks in averages, months to years. Years. A lifetime. Your life will never be the same once that baby comes, people said when they saw my pregnant belly. My life will never be the same.

First published on Glow in the Woods on 6/11/13

Miss Stein Shows a Way
Tara Hart

There is a sense of something happening and there is happiness — and then it happens — sudden and soon. It happens suddenly and it is suddenly happening too soon. Suddenly there is almost not a mother. There is a lot of sudden happening and then there is a mother and there is a daughter. A small daughter a very small daughter suddenly too soon. Too small and all of a sudden there is a mother but it is too soon for feeling. It is too soon and sudden for feeling but for feeling brave and being there there all of the time there is a father. There is a father a father is there all of the time and her father is there and her mother and then his brother and his mother too. They are there with the small daughter while the sudden mother remembers what is feeling. What is being there being back there in the world after almost not being. To remember there is doing. Feeling and being there all there is too soon but there is doing doing things to feed and to plan. So there is a mother planning and there is a mother pumping and the freezing and the planning for when there can be feeding and being there all there and not frozen.

There is doing and planning and suddenly there is sickness and still too small too small for sickness. She is still too small and sick and there is the only the sudden sickness and the racing there and the prayer the prayer that went nowhere for there was then only the holding and only the dying. The feeling comes suddenly then the feeling of not happening. The feeling happens suddenly while there is holding and all is too small except for feeling. All is small beside the dying.

There is no feeling there feeling is all here and sudden as it always was here and too big for being. The smallest one gives the biggest feeling and then there was no room for anything any thing but feeling. How it happens a mother and the child still, the still child, suddenly not there. With the child not there there is still a mother feeling as it happens. There is a feeling there always there and suddenly again and again and not small. All is small beside the dying. As it happens all is small beside the holding and the dying and then the suddenly not there. The stillness. The feeling. The feeling is not small. The feeling is always here, as it happens.

Published 2012 in <u>The Colors of Absence</u>, chapbook

This is about me.

Catherine Bayly

This is about me.
This is about feeling too deeply.
This is about loving too hard.
This is about wanting something too badly.
This is about the taste it leaves in your mouth.
This is about swallowing it.
This is about living.
This is about rushing on hot coals.
This is about tripping over a chance.
This is about a scar from hot concrete.
This is about being ripped open by my heart.
This is about the dead places inside me.
This is about sprinkling water on a frying pan.
This is about watching it dance.
This is about flecks of broken womb.
This is about trees dead for winter.
This is about the gray field of tiny, halted stumps.
This is about growing them for slaughter in the springtime.
This is about angels at night in the corner of the room.
This is about slivered hallucinations.
This is about lying naked on the bathroom floor.
This is about the roadmap of my body.
This is about a beautiful night of laughter.
This is about coming home to candles lit.
This is about cradling nothing.
This is about pouring hot wine in an open wound.
This is about praying to nothing to dream of something.
This is about phantom kicks.
This is about a belly still swollen.

This is about the terror of waking up each morning.
This is about being so lucky.
This is about feeling so afraid to hurt you.
This is about staying out too late.
This is about wanting so badly to be beside you.
This is about the silent stricken look on your face.
This is about not caring if you've made it this far.
This is about having a girl I call sissy.
This is about her kissing your cold cheek.
This is about a perfectly still projection.
This is about a heart that has ceased to beat.
This is about the first time I saw your face in white and black.
This is about you knowing my voice.
This is about babies feeling pain.
This is about the first time you never called me mama.
This is about "getting out".
This is about "getting over it".
This is about the eyes I knew were blue.
This is about dark hair I will only see glued to manila paper.
This is about baby feet inside of me.
This is about the baby knees I never knew.
This is about "Baby's First Christmas".
This is about the lifespan of butterflies.
This is about the locket I grab when I think of you.
This is about making the three of us my labor of love.
This is about seeing you trot into her room.
This is about seeing you walk out bewildered.
This is about snuggling you at night.
This is about listening for your cry in vain.
This is about time travel.
This is about present wrapping.
This is about dropping pine needles.
This is about Halloween candy.
This is about grieving alone at night.

This is about the way you hold me in the crook of your neck.
This is about quilts with your name on them.
This is about being your sweet pallbearer.
This is about being so proud of my perfect girl.
This is about our beautiful rosebud baby.
This is about starving to death.
This is about oozing deep dark red.
This is about my head on kitchen cabinets.
This is about never being the same.
This is about grasping for independence.
This is about seeing the future in a greasy skillet.
This is about a day without lavender suicide.
This is about a white dress stained always with your blood.
This is about breasts full with milk to feed you.
This is about touching feet at night.
This is about feeling you inside me.
This is about everything.
This is about nothing.
This is about green glass shattered over my crimson life
   blood.
This is about keeping you warm and full of love.
This is about your sleeping bones in the cold cold ground.
This is about knowing our picture lies with you there.
This is about all the stories I read to you.
This is about the places you'll never go.
This is about giving you life forever.
This is about a greater pain.
This is about some god needing angels.
This is about things happening for no reason.
This is about "the last mystery in obstetrics".
This is about meant to be, my baby.
This is about me not meant to be your mommy.
This is about my dead heart melting with my heavy killing
   coffin stomach.

This is about the way I love you when you touch me.

This is about your brave heart.

This is about wishing you would shrink to a size I could hold.

This is about being real.

This is about dropping to my knees on the floor.

This is about crying out for mother nature to take — me — too.

This is about knowing each day is another without your baby lips.

This is about knowing what a beautiful loving woman you would have been.

This is about not seeing you dance with your daddy.

This is about you missing a dance with your daughter on your wingtips.

This is about looking in your face and seeing her.

This is about being my own person.

This is about being broken open again.

This is about our tiny sage green dollhouse family.

This is about forever the rest of my life.

This is about choking on how much I love you.

This is about not caring if you've read to the end.

This is about me.

Untitled

Joanne Cacciatore

The rain fell
From the inside
Of the store, I saw
Monsoons intruding upon summer
Delivering fury from the heavens
Onto the asphalt

I hesitated
Should I wait out the storm?
But she has taught me
Not to wait
And what is wrong
With wet hair and sticky clothes?

And so, with intentions
Of running through the lot, safely to the car
Leaving behind the croissants and paper towels
The door opened automatically
But the plan was interrupted

She caught my eye, to the left
A mother and her little girl
She was protecting her
From the rain
She removed her coat, kindergarten-yellow
Held it over her daughter's head
She was afraid of wet hair and sticky clothes
Maybe pneumonia?
And they ran

Through the puddles, and they splashed, and they laughed
And then safely got into their car

My mind attacked me as I stood frozen on the sidewalk
I wasn't expecting the assault
Delivering fury from the Heavens
It caught me off guard and
The video rewound to August of 1994

The monsoons that fell, suddenly
Like your death
(Sorrow that intruded upon the joy of delivery)

I was watching the television
But it wasn't on
(As frequently my mind)

I rushed to the window
Rain began to pour
Like the tears, since your death
Panic struck like lightning
And as any good mother
Needing to protect her little girl
From wet hair, sticky clothes, maybe pneumonia,
Systematically, taking what I would need
To shelter her from the storm
Primary blue tarp (as an umbrella)
And a mother's heart for comfort...
But then, the shovel hidden beneath the gardening tools
Collecting dust, as her nursery
Screamed, "Take me! Save your little girl!"

I could not rescue her from the storm that day
As I tried to leave, her father pulled me from my car

25

Kicking and fighting, I protested, pleaded
But he would not allow me to go (I hated him)
To protect my child
As any good mother should

Her body, surely drenched
No splashing, no laughing
And through the night
Thoughts of wet hair, sticky clothes and pneumonia
Haunted and scorned me
Sleep does not come easy
For a mother who cannot safeguard her child

We did not get into our car, safely
I could not deliver her from death.

First published in <u>Dear Cheyenne</u> by Joanne Cacciatore
Published by MISS Foundation, Copyright 1996

Hope

Hannah Logan Morris

I know mothers who have lived a nightmare.

The mother who fears her adopted baby will be taken back.

The one who waits and waits and no adoption ever comes
  through.

The mother whose baby never wakes in the crib.

The one whose baby dies in childbirth.

And others, mothers who could say, "I am a mother"
With no living proof.

This was my worst nightmare. For a child of mine to die.

I think about my ancestors, those strong Nebraska farmwives,
  those unknown Texas
housewives, who watched baby after baby, child after child,
  succumb to all
the fragile limits of mortality.

Now I have a new nightmare—that theirs could become
my own, one more stone on my chest.

I hope this is the only worst day of your life, my mother
  wishes me, on the day
I give birth to our baby boy
who had already died.

Published on "These are the things I'm made of" 4/17/13

Below, Beneath, Beside

Tara Hart

When she died, we found the Pope had saved
a place for us to fall backwards, folding at the knees.
We'd parsed the high-browed tightrope for years, grieving
our mothers and those sisters who lit candles in the
seasons as well as in ordinary time.
Then she was swept away from us, left us startled
spiders in the empty corners of our new rooms
trying to breathe, to spin without silk.
But someone knew someone who knew
a priest and this we knew how to do: to call him Father,
to make coffee, to gather at the round dining room table,
and my mother chose hymns of wings, eagles and angels.
It would all be a bedspring, give a way of being for a while.
Calls could be made and flowers would know where to take
their fragrant faces, we remembered the words and kneeling
places, the church was full and my two brothers were more
than enough to shoulder the tiniest box.
It was also a door, one she pushed us through,
as if this suffering could save the world.

Published 2012 in <u>The Colors of Absence</u>, *chapbook*

Of This We Will Not Speak.

Angie Yingst

You came into my home,
and did not speak of death.
But death was what we were doing.

We smoked it into our fallen lungs,
puffed it out until it hung in rings above our head.
We leaked it from our unused breasts until it pooled
  below us.
We ate stillbirth for brunch with runny quiche.
We sipped on eulogies, written in deep merlot ink.
We shat bills for cremation services and grief counseling.
We collected tears,
  a brackish grey water system for our memorial gardens

You said that death talk made you uncomfortable.
And besides, you said, you wouldn't want to talk of death, if
  your baby died.

I thought that I would call you again
when I could speak of something other than death.

I still think that some days.

This piece was originally published in the chapbook, <u>Of This, We Will Not Speak</u>. Charleston, SC, CreateSpace Independent Publishing Platform (December 3, 2011).

Untitled

Catherine Bayly

Walking on pavement after some early storm, over blown
  leaves from trees,
still, with striations of green and wick at their stems, in
  brilliant reds and
  yellows that feel too vivid and young to have fallen,
  unaged and ageless—
I've wailed they should be brown, withered, crumbling
  easy to whitish dust;
their hushed youth welling up inside me, a reflection of
  myself and the eyes
of children who sing loud with pliant, cherry fleshed
  mouths—stepping into
one of those miraculous small tornadoes, I've stood at its
  center, all warm wind,
while the crimson, gilt, and evergreen swirled up around
  me, dazzling my eyes.

Spoiled Epiphanies (or, when the poet is broken)
Beth Morey

I sit here in the dark
night of my own raw
  soul and
pretend that I know what I am doing
  here, dragging
  ink across the skin
  of fallen trees, as if
the questions I bleed
have answers.

what is poetry if not seeing
  and feeling,
    and feeling, feelings
  running deep
and okay – do I see, notice
  the gray pigeon feathers that heave
  by on drafts of passing
  cars reeking, leaking gasoline fumes
and okay – do I feel?

  oh, I've felt it all, the feeling
it lays thick

over this heart like
a callous that is not protecting,
  not healing, not
  a callous
    at all.
death and birth and

all that falls in the fleeting gasp of breath, oh
    I have known you
        too well
        too well.

what
does this pen run
with if not the amniotic rush
of learning all this hushed
    and holy heart-breaking-open
and standing witness
    to my own golden, squalid, spoiled
    incense-scented epiphanies?

I sit here, in the dim
iron excavation of the soul (it heals,
    I'm told) and
trust that I am – we
are all – I am
    I am
        doing the best I can.

Stillborn, adj.
Catherine Bayly

One week later, I looked up stillborn.
Feeling too done-before, and shocking
in its frequency, and like a dirty word
that was something that described us,
science or statistics that made my mouth
constrict and then soften with moisture.

I went to the library to do it, feeling
guilty and disgusted reading about
myself in my own dictionary, but
theirs was great yellowed white,
crackling pages, millions of words
and people looking for themselves

there, I found a moth pressed
between the pages, like its own
little translucent, ephemeral leaf,
with veins for words, and blood
drained out, and more years dead
than living, and through its forewing

I read *(of an infant) born dead.*

Thank You Notes

Tara Hart

For the foothold for a while, in the other world,
even when the straddle cracked my sternum, and my
eyes, wearing white, almost drowning in the river, saw
truth in every face. My tongue tasted blood from what
everyone bit back, but I can't stop walking, wanting
back in.

For letting your grandmother hear your voice that time
she was afraid.
She'll go before me to hold you, and this is a helpful idea,
as are the colors your absence gives to the sky.

For sending that dream, the one where I wake and
am ready,
bristled with the quills and feathers of a sordid poet,
crackling with grace, finding in my own flesh
and the hard earth that cannot ground you
cloudless ways to say what you mean

Published 2012 in The Colors of Absence, chapbook

Love Notes for Lost Babies

Catherine Bayly

We are rolling scrawled notes into finger length tube shapes,
    and, trembling,
we stuff them into limp balloons, waiting to be filled with
    helium and sent
above trees, into sky full of clouds where my Eleanor sees
    parrot-shapes, worries
they might fly off—then her small voice, *Sometimes you
    have to let them go.*

There is a woman listening—my eyes are everywhere
    between glances at her—
she is lying in a man's arms, wearing tough fingerless
    gloves—but Eleanor's
breathing and laughter like bells bend her in ways a body
    shouldn't bend—
she folds against him like a kept note—halving down to
    nothing with ease
under black coats, hiding her soft stomach and big breasts
    like secrets inside.

Letters like the one in my hand, words crafted in quiet times
    I've wished for,
say it nothing like her new body screams it, folds it up and
    grows older each day
around it—right now I need the mother of her in my hands,
    scooping her folds
to build into shapes, an origami heart and a memory
    clenched inside her—

to press as flowers moments inside her pages—round legs or
   heart beating—

a pretty baby. Eleanor is dancing and they come around
   now, rolling tanks of helium,
and when they fill the space around our words—less than air
   somehow—the woman
bleats a sudden cry and it rises up with open hands that
   shock and stretch layers, up
with my noises hushed by time, up with the green balloons—
   all of them disappearing.

I'm Sorry I Forgot You.

Angie Yingst

I made your death about me.
My mistakes. My karma. My deflated belly.
My dead daughter. My goddamned fucking grief.
Perhaps the five buck fortune teller was right,
Maybe you lived your heartbreakingly short life exactly as it
was supposed to be lived.
Maybe you really are a Buddha, just like she said.
Maybe this was your last life.
And those other explanations I came up with about how you
were taken away because I didn't deserve happiness really
were big fat stupid lies that I have been hearing for a very
long time.

I have a cramped heart and a stiff soul from sitting in
meditation sitting with this grief.

I once read that the soul is like a raindrop, and when you
achieve enlightenment, you fall into the ocean. Still you,
yes, but part of something powerful and inseparable from
everything
But I want you to drench only me, Daughter. I hate the sea.
In the periodic table of elements that makes up my life now,
you are the first element. The most basic parts of nature
(regret and grief) are O+U+I.
In its most basic form, they are the weight of all sadness, and
love.

When you, my little neutron, hit my nucleus, there was
fission.

Now I am radioactive and unstable.
Your half life really was your full life.
I did it again. I made your death about me.
I am sorry I forgot you.

This piece was originally published in the hand-painted artist journal of Angie Yingst, featured in the Sketchbook Project, 2011. It is housed at the Brooklyn Art Library, both analog and digitally. Additionally, it was published in the chapbook, Of This, We Will Not Speak. Charleston, SC, CreateSpace Independent Publishing Platform (December 3, 2011).

Untitled I

Stephanie Paige Cole

What would you have done differently she asks, *if you could
    go back?*
He closes his eyes tightly, trapping hot tears
He swallows hard
She shouldn't have asked
He's reliving it now
He didn't want to
He wanted to watch TV
It has been years
He shakes his head *no.*

The puppy whines at the door and he's sure that dog is a
    saint
He touches her arm as he leaves the room
You can't go back, there's nothing you could have done
He grabs the leash and walks out the door
She closes her eyes, drifts back to that sad winter
She doesn't go back as far as he does
She knows she cannot save her
She just wants to see her
Feel the weight of her baby back in her arms
She sighs just a little as she answers her own question
More kisses, more photos, more time

Every Morning
Hannah Logan Morris

I sang to you every morning.

I
rubbed circles of lotion into my belly,
caressed my belly,
held it,
hugged it,
rested my hands on it,
gazed at it,
watched my profile in the mirror
growing.

I showed you off even though you weren't even born.

I
fed you
cheese quesadillas,
keifer,
yogurt,
ice cream,
peanut butter and jelly,
Philly cheese steaks,
rotisserie chickens and
potatoes—
mashed potatoes,
baked potatoes,
roasted potatoes.

I measured you against a list of fruits and vegetables of increasing size.

I
talked to you
in Spanish,
hugged you,
held you,
poked you,
pressed your
bottom or
feet or
head,
waited for you to
kick and
wiggle and
turn and
try to escape from my belly,
pushing out sideways up near my ribs.

I cradled you in one arm at night as I fell asleep.

And I sang to you every morning.

Published on "These are the things I'm made of" 3/30/13

The Physics of Losing You
Anne Morris

Law.
Not human laws—necessary, breakable—
but Universal.
Fact.

An object in motion stays in motion

You were moving, all the time.
Somersaults, kicks, full body rolls.
And for us, life was surging ahead,
each day closer to meeting you,
each day closer to the rest of our lives,
all the momentum of motherhood.

And then—stop.
Your heart.
Our hearts, our future.
Our baby, no longer in motion.

Our baby, breaking the laws of the universe.

(How conveniently I forget the second part,
even now whispering it under my breath:
…unless acted upon by an outside force.

Not a car crash, not the germ of infection,
not the thundering hand of God.

For you, not external but internal,
a fatal twist
a cruel accident from inside the womb.)
An object at rest stays at rest.

The tiny circle of your heart, so still.
So still and silent that not even the force
of our prayers, our screams, our love,
our labor
could move you again.

Dear baby, breaking the laws of our universe.

Transition

Kara L.C. Jones

Transition, she said.
I slid away to make the change
and the glass box around me shattered.

A million little pieces,
glistening, glinting, capturing
the face of the sun.

In this new open beauty,
I would have to re-member
myself, my body, my being.
I would have to re-wire
the motor that drives me
to veer away from constant work,
toward the pace of feet in nature,
once a day
in nature
at least.

And in the re-membering
a re-creation started.
My blood began to crawl
under my skin
with more and more agitation
until I found the foot path each day.

I remembered people talking about Peace Pilgrim.
As if her walking were *just* a recreational activity.
But in truth, it was a re-creation of self and being.

In my blood I could understand that now.

In every shard and every drop of being,
I could understand the re-creation of self in nature.

Regarding How She Is
Tara Hart

There is dozing all day, dreaming
of what might have been done.
Tears are redundant under
running water.

Grief means stuck. It has heavy
breasts, and dreads
the fragility of a crocus.

It wears a raw throat in a tight soft collar,
and wants to kill the stranger in the store
who snaps at her children.

Given the way the ground fell here,
tsunamis on the other side of the world
are perfect.

Water, milk, and blood have come
to all the ledges of me, and they are jumping.
Jumping.

I can only lie on my round softening
side, like the pear I mean to paint,
like a candle wick catching its breath,
learning to be light.

Published 2012 in <u>The Colors of Absence</u>, *chapbook*

After

Kara LC Jones

The only thing left standing,
Solid rock, heavier than God,
A statue of Jizo.

Amid the ruins of tsunami slung mud,
Ravaged garden hoses and crushed houses,
The only thing left standing.

Heavier than God,
Ravaged garden hoses and crushed houses,
A statue of Jizo, solid rock.

Solid rock, amid the ruins of tsunami slung mud,
A statue of Jizo, ravaged garden hoses, crushed houses.
The only thing left standing.
Heavier than God.

Seed of Grapefruit

Kara LC Jones

It grew in her pockets,
in the seams of her dress,
from the roots of her eyelashes,
from the valves of her heart.

A thick skin
covering a hybrid of tender pulp,
sectioned and put on display.
Some people ate, some mashed, some tried to preserve her.

The juice from seed.
The pulp from seed.
The skin from seed.
More seeds from seed.

The shaker is full of dust and air,
add ice cubes
and try not to bruise her.

I am. Still.

Angie Yingst

I am a woman whose daughter has died.
I imagined a thousand different lives she could have lived.
I imagined myself an old mother of two strong women.
I imagined our house happy.
I imagined her smiling.
I imagined her.

I am a woman whose daughter has died.
I listen to the same depressing song over and over again.
I paint maudlin pictures.
I soak in long sobbing hot baths.
I find comfort in wallowing.
I wallow.

I am a woman whose daughter has died.
I don't want to smile to make you more comfortable.
I don't want to talk about the weather with you.
I don't want to feel beautiful.
I don't want to flirt.
I don't want to comfort you.

I am a woman whose daughter has died.
She never kissed an anxious boy in an orchard.
She never fought me.
She never loved.
She never breathed.
She never.

I am a woman whose daughter has died.
I am a woman who had a daughter.
I am a woman now.
I am.

This piece was originally published on on-line poetry magazine Literary Mama, October 2009. Additionally, this piece was originally published in the chapbook, Of This, We Will Not Speak. Charleston, SC, CreateSpace Independent Publishing Platform (December 3, 2011).

Untitled II

Stephanie Paige Cole

One thing they don't tell you
in those pamphlets they hand out with
pictures of butterflies and
tiny baby feet in daddy's palms
with cherry blossom sympathy
in the background is this:

You will cry for awhile
and then you will stop
and you'll get your shit together
and feel good about it, too
because you'll have let go of the guilt
at least most of the time

and then
five years later
you will sit in your car
in the dark
in the parking lot of Barnes & Noble
and you will put your forehead on the steering wheel

and you will cry
and you will cry
and you will cry

Rainbow
Beth Morey

his ribs carve delicate
about his flickering heart and
rise, fall against
my own, deep and
profound as a whale's dive,
regular as a clock. I won't
mark time with these
breaths, the shivery
waiting for an end hammering
a(nother) chink where
the fear slips in. kissing
into his soft halo of golden strands,
smelling the sweet-sour human
smell, my soul slips
off its sandals at
                    all this holy.

                              it seems impossible
                                 that we never
                                    had this
                                      with her.

Parallel Universe

Hannah Logan Morris

I live in a world where
news of a new baby is greeted
not with congratulations but
a tremble and a quick prayer.

Where a pregnant belly in a crowd is noticed
with a swell of anxiety in the throat,
an averted gaze,
hiding the Evil Eye.

In every group of children gathered I look for the missing
ones.
The one lost, perhaps, between siblings just a few extra years
apart.
I search the mothers' faces for signs,
the scars of miscarriage, infertility, stillbirth, loss.

The ground we walk is brittle and thin.
We tread gently,
yearning for babies,
afraid to hope.

Flesh and muscle
the hearts that pump our raw, fragile lives—
Laid bare.
All the skeletons visible, everyone an x-ray,
Stark black and white, empty cavities.

Everywhere are accidents.
Every new life a potential death.

Sophia

Beth Morey

i could not comprehend what
she meant, that
fellow mother, when she said
she felt a second
baby waiting,
waiting to come through
and through her womb out
into this bright and bleeding land.

"come through
what?" i asked, but
she did not say.

i could not comprehend
until, in the haphazard clutter
of a thrift shop,
  i felt her
    (i felt her),
my own unconceived one
and it was then
that I knew
for sure
that there is a space in our hearts for one
                              more.

i named her sophia then
and there in the shop and plucked
a turquoise jumper from the rack
that wept and whispered maybe. i took

it home and crushed it to my heart, soft
corduroy tear damp and tried not
to want it too much. i smoothed her
first piece of evidence into a drawer
to incubate while my husband shook
his head at all this grief-streaked hope. i

pray this not-here-yet
girl would come through
  (come through, please God)
and be the daughter we get to keep
                              this time.

In Between

Beth Morey

she slips along
the sidewalk with a belly full
of baby [again] and only poetry
books tucked up
in her arm's crook and
she prays to feel powerful
as if God has sung silent
words into her ear and all
the rattling questions are answered

now

Why I Cannot Join a Moms Group
Stephanie Paige Cole

Surrounded by women
With children in their arms
On their laps
Circling their legs

I belong and I don't

I meet the criteria to be in this club
With a little one balanced on my hip
Playing with my hair

It is a typical mom conversation
What foods have you introduced?
Is he sleeping through the night?
Anyone thinking about having a second?

That's not what's on my mind
There's a little girl laughing in the corner
She would be just her age

Now I am choking on thoughts
That I cannot turn to words
I will not allow myself to cry here

But I miss her I miss her I miss her

Talk only about the live one
You will alienate yourself
You will be the-woman-with-the-dead-baby

You will not make new friends

I repeat it until I accept it
I shut off what is real
I chat about teething
I go home and cry

Yes he's sleeping through the night
He likes pears and avocado
And we're starting to think about having another
But that would be our third.

And you don't realize how good you have it
There are things worse than sleepless nights
with cranky infants

There are sleepless nights alone

First published in <u>*Still: a collection of honest artwork & writings from the heart of a grieving mother*</u> *by Stephanie Paige Cole. Eloquent Books, Copyright 2010*

In the Sun

Kara LC Jones

Bleached skull, staring back,
empty eyes taking in life,
hungry ghosts all 'round.

Offerings made, left untouched
as death cannot be sated.

Hawk Son

Amy McCarter

Beloved hawk son
forever my muse, take flight
blue sky of my soul

Fall

Stephanie Paige Cole

I imagine you here
your birthday approaching
my heart unbroken
our family whole

the world still growing
darker and colder
but only because
it is fall

Death is No Thing

Catherine Bayly

I sit on the deck, and the silence taken off from a breeze
    brushes my cheek.
I must be cubbied just so beneath the eaves of the house.
It is not nothing, cannot be nothing, there is something in
    that stillness.
Something warm and static, the negative space
That defines the small and large things that I am.

Cradling and holding up my face, the air all around me.

I get up and walk to the house, having to pull hard on the
    sliding glass door.
It must need oil, but I still don't do those kinds of things.
And I let up when the space is just large enough to pass
    through,
The relief in my neck and shoulders is immense,
Inaudible—that lack of tension is something too.

The moment after I crack my back is one of our greatest
    times.

I pour a cup of coffee, but like it lukewarm, so it's way too
    hot for drinking.
In the minutes I wait, steam pouring from the mug,
You are there--in the time I am forced to accept my own
    silence, and my moments
Ticking by, and how freshness rubs me the wrong way.
I curl my paws around the steam, hot and vital.

But I prefer the outsides of my hands, the bony crust left to
motionless room air.

Waking Up
Kara L.C. Jones

In the waking,
I looked up and saw
one stream of smoke,
not cloud,
screaming from the top of the mountain.

A celebratory ribbon,
stretched across the sky,
rock holding it down at one end,
wind streaming it from the other end.

The face of the mountain
danced in light and shadow,
sun playing with the depth & breadth of rock,
a tree here, a shrub there,
everything growing out of rock.

I closed my eyes and imagined
what will it be like when my body crumbles back to rock
    and dust.
I expected to be scared, but I was not.
Instead the visual of it came with a huge release of joy,
a relaxation of being I'd never known,
a falling away of the fragile container,
to be streamed across the sky and sun,
the wind carrying what was once "me,"
what now was All And Nothing.

Winter

Stephanie Paige Cole

the coldness creeps in
and my body remembers
winter is so hard

Broken hearts and a little blue dress
Stephanie Paige Cole

Innocently I pulled back the lid
and years of dreams,
broken hearts and a little blue dress
leaped out like lions
and ripped into my soul.

So much time had passed
since I'd touched that fabric,
the proof of what was surely about to be
but then wasn't,
that it sucked the breath out of my lungs
and left me shaking.

Pink snowsuit with bunny ears
and an orange sundress
shouted out that you were real. Human.
Not just an idea or an inspiration,
a daughter.
And it broke me all over again.

I dream of you constantly,
pretty little girl with deep brown eyes,
you are in the very marrow of my bones
but today I was reminded
by a little blue dress
that you were more than dreams
and it crushed me.

(The dress has been folded, it is back in the box.
The lid has been replaced.
But I can't shake these thoughts of what almost was,
and I am not okay.)

Roses and Stuffing

Catherine Bayly

How do you keep collecting things.
Maybe it's part of the magic of mothering you.
I live through the barrel of stuffed animals
that smell new and lightly dusty, and not like you at all.

You smelled like a rose cut days ago.
And your skin was just as soft.
And kissing you felt that way too.
Not like the plush horse in the nursery.
But cool and smooth, I would drink you in again.

Now I sift through packages and old cards,
Once upon a time sorted in two piles:
A small stack of congratulations
and too many sympathy cards to read at once.
Dried roses I got to keep and a dusty mobile of stuffed bugs.

Love Brings Hope and Life

Sherokee Ilse

It begins with deep, abiding love
Wanting more, waiting for new life
Planning for a future forever changed with
Children.

Then suddenly lightning strikes
Followed by a deep, lonely
Darkness
.

Who could be prepared
For this type of anguish?
So alone, yet trying to be
Together.

Love pulls us through
Each day as we struggle to
Survive.

Head down, heart broken,
Stress and confusion
Lead to arguments, silence, and
Pain.

Glimpses of beauty
Reminders of love
Eventually bring some
Hope.

Life and time march on,
While memories remain.
We are one; we will remember.
Love reminds us to
Live—
Again.

On drowning six years later
Stephanie Paige Cole

It does not matter that I
have studied the ocean
that I know the way the
waves move
that I understand the ebb
and flow
I can anticipate the current's drag
and still drown

I wish she wasn't dead

The Migration of My Heart

Devany LeDrew

Geese calling to one another
above us they fly
in the pewter sky.

Beneath, I walk
with my two babies
always yearning for my third.

The birds
with miles traveled
are always drifting away
and falling back into formation.

Their smooth dance choreographed
by honks and calls.
Searching, checking, they migrate and return.
Their music is lonely and heartbreaking,
though they are together.
Somehow the sound comforts me.

Geese calling to one another
form a V
outlined in the gray, drab sky.
I find her there.

Dots (for Angie)

Catherine Bayly

There is something about a dot,
on your clothes, on paper,
made by blotting a stamp
or dropping ink,
that old immutable feeling—
the moment   when something damp
sinks inside a surface
and lingers in stark singularity
against a space behind it,

yet math has studied these things
under microscopes, over time,
and somehow with
their number poems
they've said a dot
is self contained
infinity, what we laymen
see as just one thing
is more connected lines
than our brains can fling
against the sun

so math mothers see
these fragments
expand on themselves, spun
in constant, explosive bloom
that won't stop spinning—all newness and rippling—
despite what we see,
in the smallness of a dot.

And we are watching birds on a wire,
as they take off on some invisible cue
we can't pin down for all our watching and listening
so we stare as even stragglers labor off into red horizon—
and you call it a moment, *what a moment*, you say,
and we are silent as I send a message from my brain
to your brain about how those raven-black birds lift off
in lines, forever, moving from this thing we call our time—

and they've disappeared yet change the wind somewhere
with their wings and the wind
will move the trees and the trees
will drop leaves which will freeze
beneath snow which will grow
in spring, *oh*, the children will say
as they stroke new growths of earth
popping up in vast ground through holes
we see as round but they are shapely
beyond our imagination, concentric only in quick glances,
growing new lines in time,
making way for all the growing
things and freckling the earth with pox
like beauty marks.

Hawk

Amy McCarter

I do not feel alone when the hawk calls
As I lay quietly in bed, lazy with eyes half open
He calls
A smile forms upon my lips
My heart opens to love's magic.

I do not feel alone when the hawk sings his song.
As I sit in the morning stillness, wondering, wishing
I look up, always looking up, searching for what soars above.

I am not alone when the hawk calls out "I am here"

Pumpkin Patch

Amy McCarter

Dancing in the pumpkin patch
scents of Autumn surround
a little boy smiles
messy curls bouncing on his head
Running through the orange delight
giggling with excitement and joy
looking for the magic one
Found, he turns his sparkling eyes to me
I reach to hold his soft sweet hand
he is gone.

Fall inching

Catherine A.G. Bayly

It is decidedly chilly, and the light is pouring over the trees, just so. Red, bright and smoke-heavy. I step out outside for a moment, and feel the cold solid weighty truth of my feet rooted on the deck boards. There is a fist of twine sleeping in the pit of my stomach, and it sneaks upward through my esophagus, triggering my crying and choking as the days grow longer and fall inches toward me. It is still summer, but there is autumn in the air — smelling of burnt leaves and screaming out, *harvest.* I shiver in the mornings now, with anticipation. I feel an almost-intrinsic pull toward apple orchards, pumpkin patches — the reaping places of the withering season. Places that smell of apple cores, and cinnamon-rolled expanses of past. Places that remind me that death goes on in perpetuity, and cry out of the pumpkins left sad to rot on our porch late into last season. Places that remind me of the still-new, gilded gravestone, lonely bearing the name and body of my daughter. Places that remind me of a knife-sharp piercing and yet somehow serrated sadness, and the soft crackle of leaves as they drop on the small grassy spots where babies sleep away forever, amidst apartment buildings and scarecrow images marching in and out of made-identical hay maze offices. As footsteps and mothers and children and fathers and birth and dying and war and crying whip by in their frenzied timeline, I stand here amidst them all, perfectly still.

I take on this sadness. Let myself feel the red-gold dawn of the death of deciduous times. This emptiness unspeakable, as the earth turns its way toward a time when the burning leaves and last attempts at outdoor life will surely sneak their way into my room at dusk. Curl around my throat and choke me with the smoked odor of autumn roots and life's frigid certainties. My soft, wracked body is complete and dense in its sadness, as I shudder away from a leaf that gently whispers across my bare right shoulder on its descent to the purple, climbing earthfloor. I sob silently while my teeth are chattering, and there is the faint and imagined odor of pumpkin pie on the air as my shoulders heave in the privacy of early morning.

January

Stephanie Paige Cole

Cold and complicated
You hold within your grip
the best and worst that life has to offer
Death, birth
In that twisted order
I curse you for your cruelty
and bow down to your beauty
I beg you to be gentle with me
You break me every time.

Another Ordinary Day

Catherine Bayly

Fearing worst snow that falls without accumulation,
I press flat against the bed and watch it floating
past the trees, smoking house across the street,
toward the ground where, when lying,
                                        I envision piles
congealing into frozen, fat, epidermis, making earth
its roiling innards and covering the rush of putrid
warmth and strength, I constantly question—
what does it mean to watch it fall and disappear
into the grass, where I toss roaches and bits
of scribbled on paper from the car, that I
shuffle with the toe of laced up boots,
and where I've stretched flat, too, staring up
after driving home in falling snow to silencing
when flakes meet the ground with hisses,
and turn to nothing,
                            ratcheted down but still
like a splash inside a frying pan—where
I cook things like mushrooms that need
moisture that's settling into the bases
of trees and remaining invisibly there, and
I taste warm decay and they slide past my lips—
like the moment you have something and
then you don't, a comic explosion of stars
and onomatopoetic pff when your sandwich
is gone from the fridge or your baby dies
or a star that might as well have been our
sun is said to have fizzled out in some

other galaxy, and it is too much to accept
that some snow is zapped before it's ever
stuck to anything, and I'd rather strangle
in blankets than listen to the hissing as our
pregnant hopes of fires and running out
of food give way to another ordinary day.

I dreamed you were the sun

Stephanie Paige Cole

I dreamed of you once
raven haired child with
laughing brown eyes
you are the moon
white full and watching
illuminating the world
but not quite enough
you aren't the way you
were in my dreams

I dreamed you were the sun

It's all an experiment in free form

Kara LC Jones

Staring at the rocks and dead agave plants.
Pins and needles of the agave spines protruding from sinewy
　skeletal remains.
Rubble of broken hearted stones scattered everywhere.
Sun beating down, mid-day, even the coyote don't come out
　to play.

In whatever shade we can find,
we sit and long for a heat that won't burn,
long to feel the wind, cold and bearing down,
even as the sun scorches all that is outside the tree's
　umbrella.

Seems the thirst is never quenched.
Maybe that's the experiment.
Incarnate here. Feel the full body and weight of rocks,
the tough skin stretched thin and made vulnerable
over a bone structure called man.

We think we are invincible.
We think we have such advancement.
We think we know something, anything, everything.
And yet death still trumps.
For all the living we do, death will come,
snapping each bone till the marrow
leaches out
leaving what was once alive,
spilled on sand,
bleaching in the deadly sun,

85

till all that's left are pins and needles of a spine,
protruding from a sinewy remain.
These are the things we find in the desert.
These are the ingredients of a life lived till death.
These are the frames in which we hang ourselves.
These are the needed ingredients when experimentally
cooking up a life.
These are the boundaries we push by simply cheating death
each wide eyed morning.

Objects

Angie Yingst

Above the drawer labeled
"Objects extracted from people's throats"
sat someone else's children in yellow fluid.
Lined up, the children without breath.

Tossing aside petticoats
and other symbols of a youth-imagined beauty,
the daughter poses,
hands crossed against the glass.
Unlike the other babies,
who thought they had to float lifeless,
she sent a wind to wander the halls,
blowing doors open,
menacing the cats who kept the mice at bay.

Tiptoeing around the wax models of skin disease,
on the shelf lined with other children,
a girl, once loved in idea as much as flesh,
bathed in formaldehyde.
Quietly taking in the room,
she smiled at the soap lady, and
teased the wax Siamese twins
who clung to one another three different ways.
She chose her fate amongst the Victorian medical
    instruments,
extracting the teeth of a thousand pierced skulls.
Her hair looked wild,
a halo of angry black gypsy curls.
From the other side of the room,

her mother sat amongst the oddly shaped organs
And syphilitic skulls watching her live in death.
That one time, when she died,
the girl chose to become a specimen
instead of a daughter.
We stopped the clocks at 5:45
covered the mirrors with blankets.

Her mother wears somber, itchy clothes,
though people think she is an intellectual.
Keening for two years, and silent for a lifetime,
she has black crepe running through her veins,
and a sign above her heart that says,
"Protect from idle talk."
Yet when the other women see her black clothes,
they speak of their tiresome newborns,
complain of their morning sickness,
take offense at her for not attending elegant parties
with caviar and other dead babies.
Her mother wears fancy objects made of metal and hair,
wanders museums of silence and dust in search of a time
when brave daughters chose a different life
than one with her mother.

This piece was originally published on the website Kota Loss and Compassion blog. This piece was later published in the chapbook, Of This, We Will Not Speak. Charleston, SC, CreateSpace Independent Publishing Platform (December 3, 2011).

Failed Studies of Mary

Catherine Bayly

I promise I'll look at statues I said *Promise,*
as if you hadn't just said look in eyes or
maybe don't sit alone at coffee, but I'd
never promised to speak Italian, say
the only words I knew, *perso, bambina*—

so I went to a garden where people walk
without speaking, & praying hands hide
clasped, hanging straight along backs,
only untangling to lilt against a fern,
break the center of an orange, or dip
a middle finger inside a marble dish,
bringing holy water up to lips to see
how salty it might taste & find it tastes

like nothing. Every statue is a girl
with an infant's curls running over
shoulders & against the crook of arms
& centuries' weight makes my elbows
ache and biceps furl, built for this
by phantom yearning, and my fingers
twitch to touch some virgin's lips,

us both whispering *bambina*—&
I dream I take these hundred babies
home, lay them all around my house
& muse upon their plumpness white
as bone & leave their mothers locked

in chiseled stone with sagging blades
of shoulders like this one that stands

in the garden's center, fingers spread
& palms like broken cups, I break
my prayer & bring mine up, repent
to her by stroking deep groove cut
by nothing's weight—so I sketch
the slackened bow of flesh, to remind
me later I can show you maps of *perso.*

This piece was originally published in Stealing Time Maga-
zine.

Lines Along a Womb

Tara Hart

I offered a red apple today to a
pregnant friend, and bit one myself.
Felt you show up, old sister, the way
you'd twist hard back into shape,
right on cue. You got so tough
from two sections it took hours
to get the last one out.

Tubes are not tied in bows. They cut
them, burn the ends, cinch
twice. I feel sorry for my body now
when it bleeds. What can any body
know about lines in the dark, casting
them out, about what is or is
not getting through.

Maybe I am the one not getting
the message. You keep sending the slippery
signals, the salt, the dreams.
So much, and little earlier every time.
I need some words to know what you are
thinking will happen now, sister, soldier,
what, my hero, you want to happen next.

Published 2012 in <u>The Colors of Absence</u>, chapbook

Break

Tara Hart

It is your turn to tuck and tell stories
so I let a walk take me within call. We had less
than nothing, and now we have everything.
We turn our whole bodies to the tasks of
deserving him. We do not sleep.

We too are newish born, or at least uncertain of
what to do with our hands in this world. Our old tongues
   feel
to have fallen out. We gape. We wonder what we're growing,
and for how long.

First star I greet with a hard wish from the chest
for something to break between us like a morning
meal, warm soda bread and butter, to re-seed these
bodies with our histories of how we do.

There is a thin and edgy moon: Goodnight.
In this great green room, there is a telephone,
but I don't know any more how to place the call.

It is dark and time for the dishes we will dry tenderly, leaving
little fingers of space. I listen for what I can hear towards
   home.
For now just the silence of one cricket thinking of singing,
rubbing resin, up and down, up and down, her bow.

Published 2012 in <u>The Colors of Absence</u>, chapbook

Stir

Catherine Bayly

Late at night and still we stand here
silent, our legs tangled and your arms
around my hips that touch the counter;
the kitchen is warm, smells like yeast,
careless, effervescent, rising all day
to a plump white round I dimple with a knuckle
once like a stomach that empties at my touch,
then all my fingers play along and stroke it,
collapsed to smallness, flat, fat, creamy pad.

Flour from kneading on my hands, my back is cold
now that you alternate between violin and piano,
Play something and it repeats, bittersweet with flats,
and trills up high like chimes, *no*, more like bells
in our world of winter silence slicing slow
like bows across our necks as we envy sky
giving birth to snow, and I press the dough smooth
like two wings, ovals that explode with spreading
fingers until I pool it up and punch it flat.

Watching windows for fragile-magic reasons
to do just what we do, I see you—reflected
among golden lights, swarms of wire ornaments,
bulbs and butterflies clipped to boughs,
suspended years in flight, while beyond our
grasp or sight, is some, small, stir life—
curled over the piano, and I chase bubbles
in the dough like your hands on the keys,
left crossing right in a tag-dance, and freezing
in place, lingering on one note so long.

Hours Passed

Stephanie Paige Cole

She woke up
Put her hand to her belly, smiled
He rolled over and put his hand beside hers
Well hello
Their hands followed movements from one side to another
They guessed at arms and legs
Hours passed
The happiest ones of their lives

She woke up
Put her hand to her belly
It was late, all was quiet
Her blood turned to ice in her veins
For just a moment, both their hearts had stopped beating

She woke up
Put her hand to her belly
It was a reflex, it was a mistake
It sank deeply into loose skin
Her lungs caved in
He rolled over and put his hand beside hers
They held that sad deflated dream belly

And hours passed

Wait and Collect

Catherine Bayly

Collecting carcasses of butterflies from swingsets,
and cupping them home in trembling palms,
I crucify them on sheets of scrap velvet, black
and textured with imprints of their sisters' spans

that my hands have turned to dust with stroking,
and I wear a strip of glass that magnifies, blasts
an image at my eyes when I turn my head
and one furry thorax, stretched like a Christ belly,

is close enough to disappear inside my throat
as I gasp, *Jesus*, and go back to stringing one up
by a hook on the ceiling.
                              Standing in the doorway
to my study, you watch them twirl as I tool
over a marigold cadaver, stretching its wings

that held wind yesterday and staking it down
with pins that I pluck from a dusty bassinet
that you built, that's waited years for the heft
of warm child, and that I stained with my hands,

faded flesh file of my prints catacombs now
of dust, scales, and fragile bones, and you
too say *Jesus* and *I brought your lunch* and
you have to eat it and *we're still young.*

This piece was originally published in Little Patuxent Review.

95

Not Self

Kara LC Jones

Let go the small things
skin cells finger nails salt tears
none are truly you

let rise the unseen being
thoughts, hearts, the intangible.

Waiting for Farrah

Catherine Bayly

In the year after I lost Sophie
I imagined all my pregnant friends
phoning me to say they'd lost
their babies too, how, visiting hospital
rooms on other floors, I would
hold them firmly like refluxed newborns,
upright, and I'd rub their backs,
and tell them *Oh sweet friend,*
Oh I understand and they would trust me,

                   then I would cringe,
feeling cruel and fraudulent,
as if I were inviting death to their wombs
with a crooked finger and sweet condolence—
oh, I promise I've never wished a fetus
harm, but imagining felt dangerously
close to willing, the way I'd tingle hearing
SIDS or miscarriage or begin to shake
when told of urgent prenatal visits,
always with fear but still—my baby was

gone, so I was lonely in my house, and
I am older now, more mature, so I delight in
pregnant bellies, babies, their gurgling, impotent,
uncompromising needs, even their
bunched up rosebud lips and heads of thick
black hair, but the morbid curiosity comes up
in stranger times—a nest of birds I need too
badly to live through a storm and check with

97

unnecessary frequency, the too direct look
at the eyes of women in the park when I
mention a friend's miscarriage, hope-dreading
we will spill the contents of our hearts on
picnic tables and etch a family tree with large
chinks for lost babies, visiting a pregnant mare
and imagining her side is too still to be full
of living foal legs, telling her what I can't tell

the aging pregnant women I know whose arms
may never hold a motionless child—in that
robin's egg bank barn, dark, and half buried
in cool earth, with snake skins and hay smell,
where the mare stands, huge and lazy, awaiting
the foal her owner has named Farrah, who I'm sure
each day I will find dropped but unmoving—
Oh sweet friend, Oh I understand I say
                    as I stroke her white star.

Something More than a Serenade

Tara Hart

After grief, after terror, here you've come, after all, my
vesper. The clasping ends of days are ours.

I hunch and steer this stroller like a stolen car
or a trolley stuffed with everything I own in this world.

Hail, night, Sir of the Second Chance.
I bow and cross this dipping bowl of streets in endful light.

My son's eyes are cups of trees. Here, a draught of sky.
My moonish, waxing heart.

Published 2012 in <u>The Colors of Absence</u>, chapbook

A Minute Away in Leaves
(or Grief, seven years after losing Sophie)
Catherine Bayly

Walking straight away, toward a field of grass
carpeted by curled carcasses of leaves, I see a crown
your sister made of fallen four pronged sheathes—
she tied a switch into a long round, a hoop,
slipknots, all along it, strung with crunching
remains of the silver-black maple

in the center of our yard,
where I find I'm sitting on wet ground,
forgetting about my escape or wanting a minute away
from noise, because almost dreadfully there is no noise at
    all,
so still just beyond the walls of the house, where our electric
bodies hum, consume, make static with dancing, having not
    yet burrowed
their way into the earth to feed the worms and grow,

oh, new things, sprouts the children call them,
that pushed themselves out from where I'm curling up now,
beneath the brown and broken, and between leaves that
I rub with my finger and thumb, as if turning pages, and
    turning
them to dust when a gentle touch feels something
too rough to be your skin—and they drop to the ground as
    lead or feathers
when it frustrates me that I can't remember your skin

which the nurse promised I'd never forget, but that skin
has been supplanted—it is their skin, it is cut roses on my
　　lips,
it is the cheek of another newborn when I close my eyes to
　　shut out difference,
it is the muzzle of a quiet horse or the way I imagine birds'
　　wings,
it is gone in these years, eaten by dark dwellers, fulfilling
some cosmic cycle of being food I can't understand,
it is somewhere in the piles of leaves—and I close my eyes
and run my fingers upward through the grass like your wild
　　black hair I clipped
and buried, until I find a soft thing and I finger its veins
and it is smooth and lightly hairy like your skin—it must
　　have been —

opening my eyes, I see I am holding a red leaf with sharp
　　green points,
blown in from a tree I don't see as I scan the street
so full of brown and gold, so full of long summer lives that
　　course
until they wither, being born then growing and then growing
　　old,
yet this natural blood colored thing feels young and warm,
　　if still, and it curls,
with velvet skin, much more delicate than the rest, into a
　　small ruby cup

Five

Stephanie Paige Cole

five years have passed
since I saw you, held you, kissed you
but I know your soul
and feel your spirit with me
Madeline, you were not lost.

Negative Spaces

Catherine Bayly

Not looking on empty playgrounds much anymore.
Smiling at sun making stripes with trees and browning leaves
    instead.
Cyclical days of sky pink and sweet music.

Blue crops up, flashing impressions of your eyes.
White clouds like corn popping, salt melting into crevices.
Stepping on crinkled, ruddy tree stars.
Photographs of the nothing between blades of grass.

Night comes on purple, then black like hair.
Morning rises like cream paper around your clippings.
Heart breaks and it breaks softly now.
Rain drops and lands by eyes and lips.
Taste and it is clear, fresh, and it hurts clean.
Chin still trembles when another girl has your name.

But I fill the spaces with anything-but peach walls
And memories built up strong like castles.
Growing older now, but peace lives in these wrinkles.

Serenity is in the Storm
Beth Morey

I always thought
that peace had to come before peace could come inside.

And so I waited
for life to assemble itself more neatly
than the hodgepodge trauma of shock and loss and tears and
    broken parts
that it is, that it seems always
to have been.

But life never does line up like I think it should
and mess upon mess is born.
I cry myself into sleep's imitation
and know that it must be me, doing it all wrong.
I am wrong.

Until
I blink my weary eyes clear enough to see
that I am not the only one who cries.

But those who weep are not all lost, trapped in the waiting
for life to bring the calm.
They weep in grief and weep in peace.
They are not broken.

I try wonder –
maybe it's the waiting that is wrong,
and not my self.

Some new truth begins to roil inside my heart, rolling in the
    muddy vessels,
something radical and brave that I never dared consider –
that maybe peace does not hang on circumstance
but can be born from within
and without:

Peace like a river, as they say, flowing from the One Who
    Made Me,
eroding the banks of fear and pain to softly wash my salt-
    stung face.
I can choose to believe,
to ride the skiff of hope built to carry me through these
    warring storms,
or not.

But if I do . . . if I do, that
is where peace takes root
and blossoms
beauty from ashes,
here.

Serenity can dwell between the thunderclaps,
and does.
I seek it there and my rattling heart grows calm.

I breathe and feel and feel and stand
to wait no more.
Peace draws near, gentle guardian in the gale.

Full Moon
Stephanie Paige Cole

On clear quiet nights
I can see her in the moon
She is beautiful.

A Beautiful Many Hanging Art
(For Stephanie Cole, January 5, 2012)

Catherine Bayly

I watched a woman hanging art today—
approximating levels and appraising light—
small like a girl with a brown shock of hair
along her spine, defiant fists of fingers
stacked on her hips, and though
I stood in a doorway facing her back,
I imagined a full moon in her neck
and her chin tipped up at jagged
red images from hoarse days,
when nothing roared loud enough,
gushed hot blood enough,
and I felt that speechless loneliness
making my insides scream, contract,
then burst and flood with sticky blood
like the gallery filled with caramel light
that smelled like a little girl's ice cream cone,
and I breathed it, gasped, and the walls peeled
with bits of tiny laughter like infinity angels
on primary xylophones and small pink tongues
and so many shades of brown hair spilling wild
out of ribbons in favorite colors locked
forever in time like something behind
her eyes that some see and others miss, and
I had to grab the doorframe because I knew
her eyes were filling and mine were filling

and that feeling in my nose and throat
like carbonation, that ephemeral swell,
and my hands on aged lengthwise grains
like stroking our inner children gone out—
when she turned to me, two hopeful smiles
like the girls we'd give our lives to see
in this honeyed light, and without the birth
of tears I imagined, she asked me
I think they're alright?
and all I could say was
I think they're beautiful.

Sacred

Stephanie Paige Cole

Your life began and
ended within my womb I
am a sacred space
because of you

Index

About the Editors

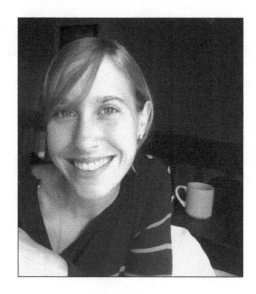

Catherine Bayly has hungrily read and written poems all her life. And writing became her constant companion and vessel after her first daughter, Sophie, was stillborn on Halloween of 2005. Since then, Catherine has published poetry, led grief writing workshops, and gotten her MA in literature. While her work has grown and changed tremendously, her children have stayed constantly at its center. Catherine now teaches writing at several lovely colleges in Maryland, where she lives with her husband and daughters. Her work can be found in *Exhale, Still Standing, Stealing Time*, and *Little Patuxent Review,* as well as on her occasional blog, *The Lifespan of Butterflies.*

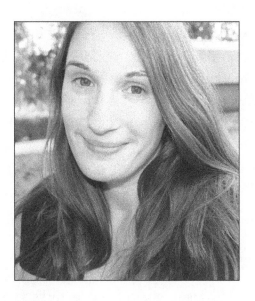

Stephanie Paige Cole has been writing ever since she learned how to spell, but never as ferociously as after the death of her firstborn child in January 2007. Born in New York City, Stephanie now resides among the farms of Lancaster County, Pennsylvania with her husband and their three sweet sons. She works at an art gallery as a writer and occasionally exhibits her own paintings, sculptures and photography. Stephanie is the author of *Still: a collection of honest artwork & writings from the heart of a grieving mother* and the founder of Sweet Pea Project, a nonprofit organization that offers comfort, support and gentle guidance to families who have experienced the death of a baby.

About the Contributors

Dr. Joanne Cacciatore is a professor and researcher at Arizona State University and the founder of the MISS Foundation, an international nonprofit organization with 75 chapters around the world aiding parents whose children have died or are dying. She is also a medical consultant and trainer who has presented grand rounds and provided individual and agency consulting and training all around the world.

Carly Dudley is an artist, photographer, public speaker, and writer from Perth Western Australia. After the stillbirth of her son in 2007, Carly began reaching out to others who had suffered the same sort of unimaginable loss. In 2008, Carly began her Project Heal mission that features a card line and special days dedicated to bereaved families such as International Bereaved Mothers and Fathers Days and August 19th — Day of Hope. Carly's articles on healing after loss are featured each month in *Still Standing Magazine*.

Tara Hart, Ph.D., won a Pushcart Prize for her poem "Patronized," published in Little Patuxent Review, and is author of a chapbook entitled *The Colors of Absence* (www.tarajhart. com). She serves as Professor of English, Arts & Humanities and Coordinator of Fine Arts and Creative Writing at Howard Community College and as Board Co-Chair of the Howard County Poetry and Literature Society (HoCoPoLitSo). She lives with her husband and two children, and in loving remembrance of Tessa Hart Horvath (October 12-17, 2004), in Columbia, Maryland.

Sherokee Ilse is a grateful mother of two living sons and three babies who she will meet again in Heaven. She is an international parent advocate/activist, trainer, speaker, president, and founder of BabiesRemembered.org and the author of 17 books and booklets including *Empty Arms: Coping with Miscarriage, Stillbirth, and Early Infant Death*. Helping families and caregivers in the baby loss world has been her passion and life's mission for the past three decades.

Kara L.C. Jones is the coach and heARTist behind Mother-Henna.com and is one of the co-creators and educators at the CreativeGriefStudio.com where she co-facilitates a 4-month certification course for helping professionals. She is mother to three dead children and has spent over 20 years exploring the alchemy of art, the Hero's Journey, narrative inquiry, and more on the quest to stay creatively agile as she lives her life in the face of death.

Devany LeDrew is an early childhood educator and blogger who writes at *www.stillplayingschool.com* about mothering all three of her children, including Violet who lived 2.5 short yet beautiful days.

Amy McCarter writes and creates art to help heal the devastating heartbreak endured after the death of her first born child Liam in 2007. Liam was born alive and perfect but died less than an hour later with no known cause. Amy lives in Chapel Hill, North Carolina with her husband Jason, their son Seamus and two dogs, Leo and Elbe.

Beth Morey is a mixed media artist and writer living in western Montana with her husband and their rainbow son. She is the owner of Epiphany Art Studio, the creator of the "Made" online course, and the author of the healing workbook, *Life After Eating Disorder*. Her words have appeared in various publications, such as *Still Standing Magazine,*

Wild Goslings, and *Disney's Family Fun.* She is an advocate for babyloss awareness and healthy grieving, and loves to meet new friends through her blog *bethmorey.com.*

Anne Morris lives in North Carolina with her wife, Hannah. She is a dancer, teacher, and Program Director for the North Carolina Dance Festival. Anne and Hannah's first child, Joseph, was stillborn at 35 weeks in December 2012.

Hannah Logan Morris is a writer, artist, and elementary teacher. Her and her wife Anne's first child, Joseph, was stillborn at 35 weeks on December 27, 2012. Hannah has recently taken over as editor of the babyloss site *Glow in the Woods.* She blogs anonymously about the loss of their son.

Laura Seftel is the author of the book *Grief Unseen: Healing Pregnancy Loss Through the Arts* (2006). She is an Art Therapist in private practice in Northampton, MA and the founder of "The Secret Club Project," a national project featuring women artists' experience of pregnancy loss.

Angie M. Yingst began writing about grief, art, religion, and parenting at her blog *still life with circles*, after the death of her second daughter. The blog was chosen in 2010, as one of the top 50 Must-Read Mom Blogs by *Parenting Magazine* and Blogher. Angie is the editor and a regular contributor at *Glow In The Woods*, a website dedicated to literary writing by parents grieving the loss of one or more babies. Angie's essay, "Mothering Grief", appears in a collection of essays about stillbirth called *They Were Still Born*, published by Rowman and Littlefield in 2010. She has a poetry chapbook called *of this, we will not speak.* She holds a B.A. in Religion from Temple University.